Best Anti-Inflammatory Diet Cookbook

Best Cookbook with Practical Recipes to Gain motivation and Cooking Healthy Food with an Anti-Inflammatory Diet

Susie Kessler

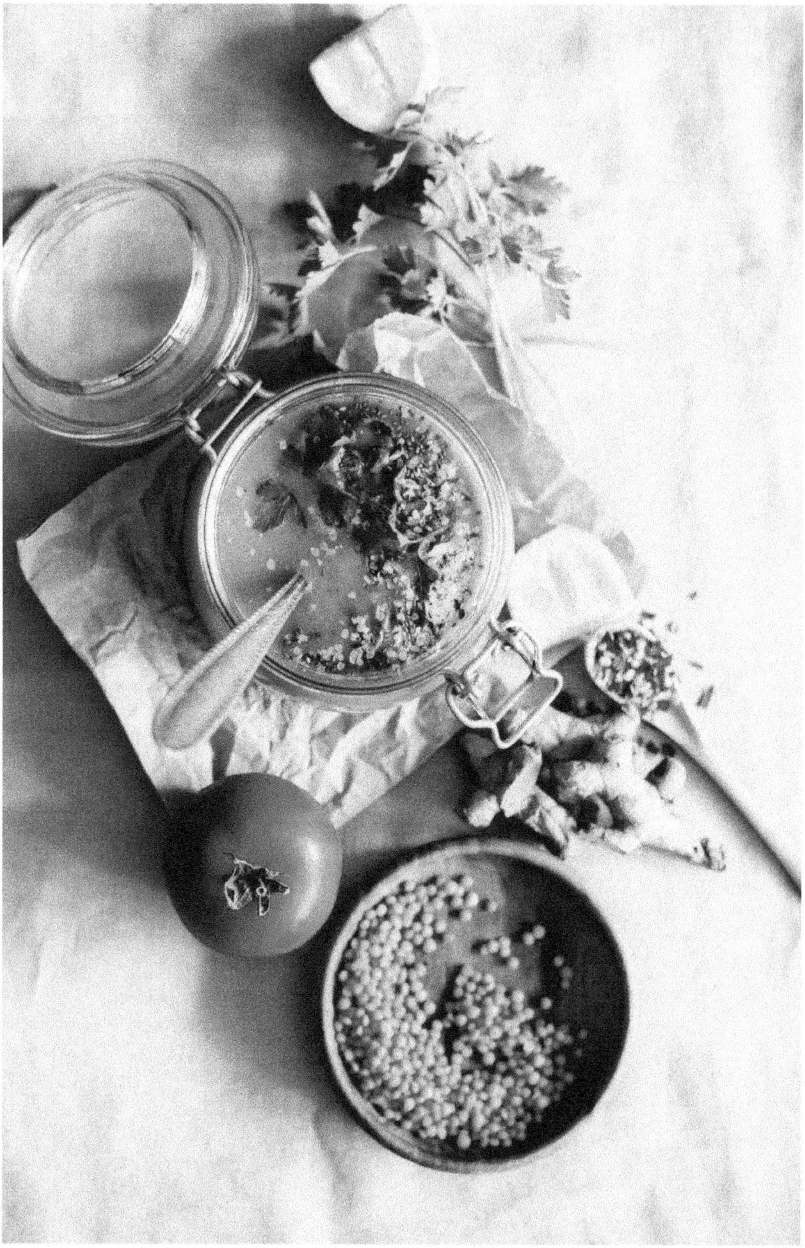

Table of Contents

broadly considered a truthful and accurate account of facts and as such, any inattention, use, or misuse of the information in question by the reader will render any resulting actions solely under their purview. There are no scenarios in which the publisher or the original author of this work can be in any fashion deemed liable for any hardship or damages that may befall them after undertaking information described herein. Additionally, the information in the following pages is intended only for informational purposes and should thus be thought of as universal. As befitting its nature, it is presented without assurance regarding its prolonged validity or interim quality. Trademarks that are mentioned are done without written consent and can in no way be considered an endorsement from the trademark holder.

Introduction

Most of the widely consumed diets incorporate anti-inflammation diet principles. In particular, the Mediterranean diet has whole grains, fish, and fats that are beneficial for the heart. Studies suggest that this diet can help lower the effects of cardiovascular system inflammation due to diet. Taking an anti-inflammatory diet is can be a complementary therapy for most conditions that are aggravated by chronic inflammation.

An anti-inflammation diet entails eating only particular kinds of food and avoiding others to lower the symptoms of chronic inflammatory diseases. It is one of the recommended measures that an individual can take to reduce or prevent inflammation induced by diet.

Expectedly, an anti-inflammatory diet involves nutrient-dense plant foods and minimizing or avoiding processed meats and foods. The goal of an anti-inflammation diet is to minimize inflammatory responses. The diet entails substituting refined foods with whole and nutrient-laden foods. Predictably, an anti-inflammation diet will contain more amounts of antioxidants that are reactive molecules in food and help reduce the number of free radicals. The free radicals are molecules in the human body that may harm cells and enhance the risk of certain diseases.

In particular, an anti-inflammation diet can help with the following diseases/conditions:

- Diabetes

Focusing exclusively on type 2 diabetes arises when the body fails to properly utilize insulin leading to higher than normal blood sugar levels. The condition of more sugar levels in the blood than normal is also known as hyperglycemia. It is also called insulin resistance. At the beginning of type 2 diabetes, the pancreas tries to make more insulin but fails to catch up with the rising blood sugar levels.

- Inflammatory bowel disease

Inflammatory bowel disease is a common gastrointestinal disorder that affects the large intestine. The symptoms of inflammatory bowel disease include abdominal pain, cramping, bloating, constipation, and diarrhea. It is a chronic condition, and it has to be managed in the long-term. Dietary measures are necessary to prevent diet-induced bloating, abdominal pain, diarrhea, and constipation. However, only a small percentage of individuals with inflammatory bowel disease will have extreme symptoms manifestation.

- Obesity

Medically, obesity refers to a complex disorder involving excessive amounts of body fat. Expectedly, obesity increases the risk of heart diseases as well as other health problems. Fortunately, modest weight loss can help halt and reverse the effects of obesity. Dietary adjustments can help address the causes of obesity, and the anti-inflammatory diet is inherently a healthy diet.

- Heart disease

Cardiovascular diseases can be triggered by diet, and diet can is used to manage several heart diseases. Food-related factors that increase the risk of heart diseases include obesity and high blood pressure. The type of fat eaten can also worsen or lesser risk of developing heart disease. In particular, cholesterol, saturated and trans fats are thought to increase heart attack rates. Most obese individuals also tend to have high-fat diets.

- Metabolic syndrome

Medically, metabolic syndrome refers to a group of factors that manifest together, leading to an increase in the risk of developing other inflammatory conditions. Some of these conditions include high blood pressure, excess body fat, especially around the waist, abnormal cholesterol, and high blood sugar levels. Having any or all of these conditions signifies that you are at a higher risk of developing a chronic condition. Most of these conditions are also associated with consuming an inflammation diet.

- Hashimoto's disease

Hashimoto's disease is an autoimmune disorder in which the body attacks its own tissues and, in particular, the thyroid organ. The result of unmanaged Hashimoto's disease is hypothyroidism implying that the body will not make adequate hormones. The thyroid gland makes hormones that control body metabolism, which includes heart rate and calories utilization. Unchecked Hashimoto's disease will also result in difficulties in swallowing when goiter manifests. Diet adjustments can be used to help manage the disease along with medications.

- Lupus

Lupus is another autoimmune disease that occurs when the body attacks its own organs and tissues. The inflammation occasioned by unmanaged lupus will affect other parts of the body. For instance, inflammation triggered by lupus will affect the heart, lungs, kidneys, and skin, including the brain and blood cells. The common symptoms of lupus are fever, fatigue, chest pain, dry eyes, and butterfly-shaped rash. Diet can be used to minimize the worsening of inflammation by adhering to the anti-inflammatory diet.

The other benefit of taking an anti-inflammation diet is that it can help lower the risk of select cancers such as colorectal cancer.

Avocado Hummus

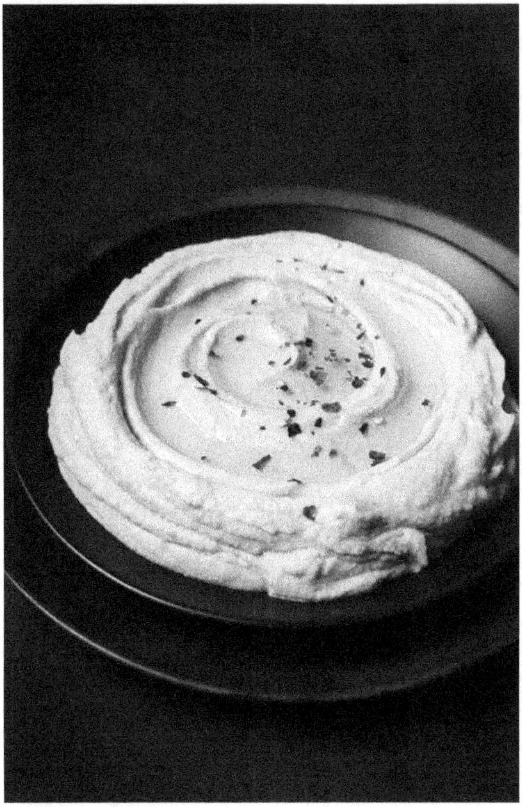

Preparation Time: 15 minutes

Cooking Time: 0 minutes

Servings: 4

Ingredients:

- .25 tsp. Pepper
- .5 tsp. Salt

- 5 tsp. Cumin
- 1 clove pressed garlic
- .5 Lemon juice
- .25 cup Tahini
- .25 cup Sunflower seeds
- .5 cup Coconut oil
- .5 cup Cilantro
- 3 Avocados

Directions:

1. Halve the avocados, take off the pits, and then spoon out the flesh.
2. Put all together ingredients in a blender and mix until completely smooth.
3. Add water, lemon juice, or oil if you need to loosen the mixture bit.

Nutrition:

Calories: 651 kcal

Protein: 9.62 g

Fat: 64.05 g

Carbohydrates: 19.95 g

Flavorsome Almonds

Preparation Time: 10 minutes

Cooking Time: 15 minutes

Servings: 8

Ingredients:

- 2 cups of whole almonds
- 3 tbsp. of raw honey
- 1 tsp. of extra-virgin olive oil
- 1 tbsp. of filtered water
- ½ tsp. of chili powder
- ½ tsp. of ground cinnamon
- ¼ tsp. of ground cumin
- ¼ tsp. of cayenne pepper
- Salt, to taste

Directions:

1. Preheat the oven to 350 degrees F.
2. Arrange the almonds onto a large rimmed baking sheet in a single layer.
3. Roast for about 10 minutes.
4. Meanwhile, in a microwave-safe bowl, add honey and microwave on Hugh for about 30 seconds.

5. Remove from microwave and stir in oil and water.
6. In a small bowl, mix together all spices.
7. Remove the almonds from the oven, add it into the bowl of honey mixture, and stir to combine well.
8. Transfer the almond mixture onto the baking sheet in a single layer.
9. Sprinkle with spice mixture evenly.
10. Roast for about 3-4 minutes.
11. Take off from oven and keep aside to cool completely before serving.
12. You can preserve these roasted almonds in an airtight jar.

Nutrition:

Calories: 168

Fat: 12.5g

Carbs: 11.8g

Protein: 5.1g

Fiber: 3.1g

Chewy Blackberry Leather

Preparation Time: 15 minutes

Cooking Time: 5-6 hours

Servings: 8

Ingredients:

- 2 cups of fresh blackberries
- 1 tbsp. of fresh mint leaves
- 1 tsp. of ground cinnamon
- 1/8 tsp. of fresh lemon juice
- ¼ cup of raw honey

Directions:

1. Set the oven to 170F. Line baking sheet with parchment paper.
2. In a food processor, put all ingredients and pulse till smooth.
3. Take the mixture onto the prepared baking sheet and, with the back of a spoon, smooth the top.
4. Bake for about 5-6 hours.
5. Cut the leather into equal-sized strips.
6. Now, roll each rectangle to make fruit rolls.

Nutrition: Calories: 49,Fat: 0.2g, Carbs: 12.5g, Protein: 0.6g, Fiber: 2.1g

Party-Time Chicken Nuggets

Preparation Time: 10 minutes

Cooking Time: 25 minutes

Servings: 6

Ingredients:

- 2 (6-ounce) grass-fed skinless, boneless chicken breasts
- 2 large organic eggs
- 1½ cups of blanched almond flour
- ½ cup tapioca flour
- ½ tsp. of paprika
- ½ tsp. of onion powder
- ½ tsp. of garlic powder
- Salt, to taste
- Freshly ground black pepper, to taste

Directions:

1. Set the oven to 400F then grease a large baking sheet.
2. With a rolling pin, roll the chicken breasts to an even thickness.
3. Cut each breast into bite-sized pieces.
4. In a shallow dish, crack the eggs and beat well.

5. In another shallow dish, mix together flours and spices.
6. Dip the chicken nuggets in beaten eggs.
7. Then roll in flour mixture completely.
8. Arrange the nuggets onto the prepared baking sheet in a single layer.
9. Bake for about 10-12 minutes, flipping once after 5 minutes.

Nutrition:

Calories: 312

Fat: 17.8g

Carbs: 15.4g

Protein: 23.6g

Fiber: 3.2g

Protein-Packed Croquettes

Preparation Time: 10 minutes

Cooking Time: 5 minutes

Servings: 12

Ingredients:

- ¼ cup plus 1 tbsp. of olive oil, divided
- ½ cup of thawed frozen peas
- 2 minced garlic cloves
- 1 cup of cooked quinoa
- 2 large peeled and mashed boiled potatoes
- ¼ cup of chopped fresh cilantro leaves
- 2 tsp. of ground cumin
- ½ tsp. of paprika
- ¼ tsp. of ground turmeric
- Salt, to taste
- Freshly ground black pepper, to taste

Directions:

1. In a frying pan, heat 1 tbsp. of oil on medium heat.
2. Add peas and garlic and sauté for about 1 minute.
3. Transfer the peas mixture into a large bowl.

4. Put remaining ingredients then mix till well combined.
5. Make equal sized oblong shaped patties from the mixture.
6. In a huge skillet, warm remaining oil on medium-high heat.
7. Add croquettes in batches and fry for about 4 minutes per side.

Nutrition:

Calories: 152

Fat: 6.9g

Carbs: 20.1g

Protein: 3.5g

Fiber: 2.9g

Energy Dates Balls

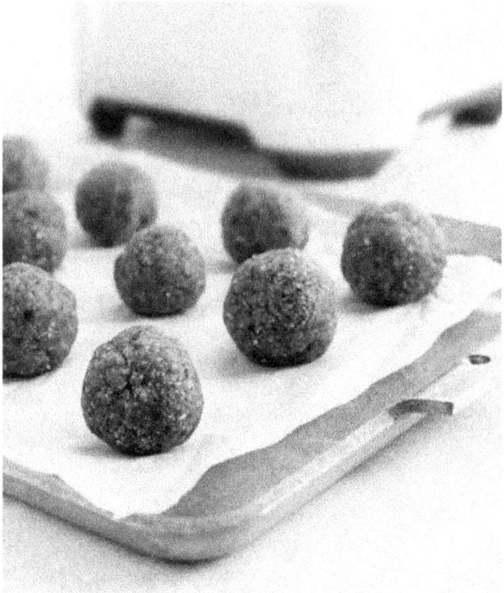

Preparation Time: 10 minutes

Cooking Time: 25 minutes

Servings: 7

Ingredients:

- 1 cup of toasted almonds
- 1 cup of pitted and chopped dates
- ¼ cup of fresh lemon juice
- ½ cup of shredded sweetened coconut

Directions:

1. Line a large baking sheet using a parchment paper. Keep aside.
2. In a food processor, add almonds and pulse till chopped coarsely.
3. Add dates and lemon juice and pulse till a soft dough forms.
4. Make equal sized balls from the mixture.
5. In a shallow, dish place shredded coconut.
6. Roll the balls in shredded coconut evenly.
7. Put the balls onto the baking sheet in a single layer.
8. Refrigerate to set completely before serving.

Nutrition:

Calories: 173

Fat: 7.9g

Carbs: 23g

Protein: 3.8g

Fiber: 4.3g

Energetic Oat Bars

Preparation Time: 10 minutes

Cooking Time: 25 minutes

Servings: 6

Ingredients:

- ½ cup of gluten-free rolled oats
- 2 tbsp. of flax seeds
- 1 tbsp. of sunflower seeds
- 1 tbsp. of chopped walnuts
- 2 tbsp. of raisins
- ¾ cup fresh blueberries
- 1 peeled and mashed banana
- 2 tbsp. of pitted and chopped finely dates
- 1 tbsp. of fresh pomegranate juice

Directions:

1. Set the oven to 350F. Lightly, oil an 8-inch baking dish.
2. In a huge mixing bowl, put all ingredients and mix till well combined.
3. Place the mixture into the prepared baking dish evenly.
4. Bake for about 25 minutes. Take off from the oven then cool.

5. Using a knife, divide the bars into the size your desired pieces then serve.

Nutrition:

Calories: 88

Fat: 2.3g

Carbs: 18.2g

Protein: 2.3g

Fiber: 2.8g

Soft Flourless Cookies

Preparation Time: 10 minutes

Cooking Time: 25 minutes

Servings: 4

Ingredients:

- ¾ cup of shredded unsweetened coconut
- 1 peeled large banana
- Pinch of ground cinnamon
- ¼ teaspoon of organic vanilla extract

Directions:

1. Set the oven to 350F. Line a cookie sheet with a large greased parchment paper.
2. In a large food processor, put all ingredients and pulse till well combined.
3. Spoon the mixture onto the prepared cookie sheet. With your hands, flatten the cookies slightly.
4. Bake for at least 25 minutes or till golden brown.

Nutrition:

Calories: 84,Fat: 5.1g,Carbs: 10.1g,Protein: 0.9g,Fiber: 2.3g

Delectable Cookies

Preparation Time: 20 minutes

Cooking Time: 15-20 minutes

Servings: 6

Ingredients:

- 1 cup of almonds
- 1 1/3 cups of almond flour
- ¼ cup of arrowroot flour
- 1 tbsp. of coconut flour
- 1 tsp. ground turmeric
- Salt, to taste
- Freshly ground black pepper, to taste
- 1 organic egg
- ¼ cup of olive oil
- 3 tbsp. of raw honey
- 1 tsp. of organic vanilla extract

Directions:

1. In a food processor, put the almonds and pulse till chopped roughly
2. Transfer the chopped almonds in a large bowl.
3. Put the flours and spices and mix well.

4. In another bowl, put the remaining ingredients then beat till well combined.
5. Place the flour mixture into the egg mixture and mix till well combined.
6. Arrange a plastic wrap over the cutting board.
7. Place the dough over the cutting board.
8. Using your hands, pat into about 1-inch thick circle.
9. Gently cut the circle in 6 wedges.
10. Set the scones onto a cookie sheet in a single layer.
11. Bake for about 15-20 minutes.

Nutrition:

Calories: 335

Fat: 27.7g

Carbs: 17.6g

Protein: 9g

Fiber: 4.8g

Turmeric Chickpea Cakes

Preparation Time: 20 minutes

Cooking Time: 30 minutes

Servings: 8

Ingredients:

- 2 small onions, minced
- 2 cans (15oz.) chickpeas, rinsed, drained
- Freshly ground pepper to taste
- 1 teaspoon cayenne pepper, to taste (optional)
- 4 cloves garlic, minced
- 4 tablespoons cornstarch
- 1 teaspoon salt or to taste
- 2 teaspoons turmeric powder
- 8-10 tablespoons chickpea flour
- Avocado dipping sauce to serve
- ½ cup fresh parsley, minced
- Grapeseed oil to fry

Directions:

1. Place a skillet over medium heat. Add a little oil. When the oil is heated, put onion and garlic and sauté until translucent. Turn off the heat and cool completely.

2. Add chickpeas into the food processor bowl and process until very finely chopped.
3. Add the onion mixture, salt, pepper, cayenne pepper, and turmeric powder and pulse again until well combined.
4. Transfer into a bowl. Add parsley and mix well.
5. Make small balls of the mixture (of about 1 inch diameter) and shape into patties. Place chickpea flour on a plate.
6. Place a nonstick pan over medium heat. Add a little oil and swirl the pan so that the oil spreads.
7. Dredge the patties in the chickpea flour and place a few on the pan. Cook in batches.
8. Cook until the underside is golden brown. Flip then cook the other side till it's golden brown.
9. Repeat steps 6-8 to fry the remaining patties.
10. Serve with avocado dipping sauce.

Nutrition:

Calories: 154 kcal

Protein: 7.32 ,Fat: 2.85 g,Carbohydrates: 25.43 g

Almonds and Blueberries Yogurt Snack

Preparation Time: 10 minutes

Cooking Time: 0 minutes

Servings: 2

Ingredients:

- 1 ½ cups nonfat Greek yogurt
- 20 almonds, chopped
- 1 cup blueberries

Directions:

1. Take 2 bowls and add ¾ cup yogurt into each bowl.
2. Divide the blueberries among the bowls and stir.
3. Sprinkle half the almonds in each bowl and serve.

Nutrition:

Calories: 223 kcal

Protein: 6.57 g

Fat: 9.45 g

Carbohydrates: 30.82 g

Peanut Butter and Honey Oat Bars

Preparation Time: 10 minutes

Cooking Time: 25 minutes

Servings: 18

Ingredients:

- ¼ cup honey
- 3 tablespoons peanut butter
- ¼ cup honey roasted peanuts, chopped
- 2 teaspoons coconut oil
- ¼ teaspoon cinnamon powder
- ¼ teaspoon vanilla extract
- 1 cup oats

Directions:

1. Line a small baking pan using a parchment paper such that the parchment paper is hanging over the sides of the baking pan.
2. Add honey, oil, and peanut butter into a microwave-safe bowl. Microwave on High for around 20 -30 seconds or until the peanut butter melts completely. If it takes longer than 30 seconds, stir and cook in increments of 10 seconds, stirring each time.

3. Take off from the microwave and add the rest of the ingredients. Mix well and pour into the prepared baking pan. Spread the mixture and press with a spatula.
4. Bake in a preheated oven 300° F for about 20 minutes or until the top is light brown.
5. Remove from the oven and press once again.
6. Cool for a while and slice.
7. Cool completely and serve.
8. Transfer leftover bars into an airtight container. Refrigerate until use.

Nutrition:

Calories: 44 kcal

Protein: 1.47 g

Fat: 1.69 g

Carbohydrates: 8.06 g

Cottage Cheese with Apple Sauce

Preparation Time: 5 minutes

Cooking Time: 0 minutes

Servings: 2

Ingredients:

- 5-6 tablespoons cottage cheese
- ½ teaspoon cinnamon powder
- 2-3 tablespoons applesauce or more if required

Directions:

1. Divide the cottage cheese into 2 bowls.
2. Spread applesauce over the cottage cheese.
3. Sprinkle ¼ teaspoon cinnamon powder on each and serve.

Nutrition:

Calories: 79 kcal

Protein: 8.09 g

Fat: 3.45 g

Carbohydrates: 3.92 g

Cucumber Rolls Hors D'oeuvres

Preparation Time: 20 minutes

Cooking Time: 0 minutes

Servings: 8-10

Ingredients:

- 2 large organic English cucumbers or 4 normal cucumbers
- For the avocado spread:
- ½ cup capers
- 1 teaspoon Himalayan pink salt
- ¼ cup fresh dill, finely chopped
- ½ cup fresh parsley + extra to garnish, finely chopped
- 5-6 ripe avocadoes, peeled, pitted, mashed
- Freshly cracked pepper to taste

Directions:

1. Peel the cucumbers and cut thin slices along the length on a mandolin slicer.
2. Place the cucumber slices on your countertop.
3. To make the avocado spread: Add all the ingredients of avocado spread into a bowl and mix until well combined.

4. Spread the avocado mixture evenly and thinly on the cucumber slices.
5. Start rolling from one of the shorter ends to the other end and place on a serving platter with its seam side facing down.
6. Repeat the above step with the remaining cucumber slices.
7. Serve immediately as the cucumbers tend to get soggy after a while.

Nutrition:

Calories: 227 kcal

Protein: 3.77 g

Fat: 19.88 g

Carbohydrates: 12.99 g

Ginger Turmeric Protein Bars

Preparation Time: 10 minutes + 20 cooling time

Cooking Time: 25 minutes

Servings: 7

Ingredients:

- ½ cup coconut
- 1 Tbsp. ginger
- 1 scoop turmeric protein bone broth
- 2 Tbsp. maple syrup
- 1/3 cup sunflower butter
- 1 cup cashews

Directions:

1. Add coconut pieces and cashews to a blender or food processor. Use the pulse option to obtain a coarse mixture.
2. Add butter, broth, maple syrup, and ginger and pulse the mixture to form a coarse, yet even and somewhat sticky mass.
3. Evenly place the mixture to a baking pan (8x8 inches) with your hands or a spoon. Push firmly to the baking pan.
4. Bring it in a refrigerator and let it cool for 20 minutes.

5. Cut the mixture into even squares.
6. You can consume immediately or store in a glass container in your fridge (up to 7 days).

Nutrition: 107 kcal

Protein: 1.15 g

Fat: 9.59 g

Carbohydrates: 4.63 g

Avocado with Tomatoes and Cucumber

Preparation Time: 10 minutes

Cooking Time: 0 minutes

Servings: 2

Ingredients:

- 2 avocados
- 1 cucumber
- 4 Roma tomatoes
- ½ red onion
- 1/8 cup parsley
- ¼ cup cilantro
- ¼ cup olives – to your choice
- 1 lemon
- 1 Tbsp. turmeric
- Salt and pepper – to your taste

Directions:

1. Dice the tomatoes, cucumber, avocado, and olives.
2. Slice the cilantro, parsley, and onion.
3. Add the above ingredients into a bowl.
4. Squeeze the lemon juice then add to the vegetables.

5. Add olive oil, turmeric, salt, and pepper.
6. Toss well.
7. Consume immediately after adding lemon juice and olive oil.
8. If you prefer to consume the salad later, add the dressing immediately before consuming it.

Nutrition:

Calories: 480 kcal

Protein: 11.57 g

Fat: 35.27 g

Carbohydrates: 39.77 g

Salmon & Avocado Toast

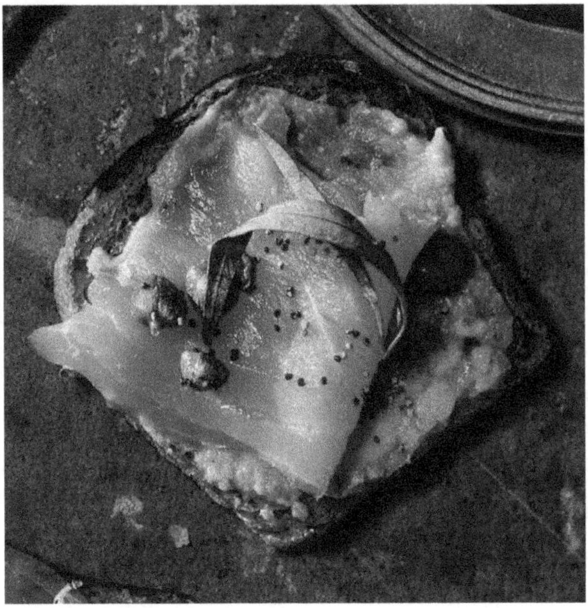

Preparation Time: 10 minutes

Cooking Time: 5 minutes

Servings: 1

Ingredients:

  - oz. pink salmon (wild)
- 2 slices of gluten-free bread
- ½ avocado
- ¼ tsp red pepper
- 1 tsp lemon juice

- salt and pepper - to taste

Directions:

1. Slice the avocado.
2. Toast the bread to your taste.
3. Mix the salmon and lemon juice.
4. When the toast is ready, lay avocado slices onto it.
5. Cover with salmon.
6. Add some red pepper, salt, and pepper to your taste.
7. Feel free to put the other ingredients you like (tomatoes, onions)
8. Enjoy your salmon snack!

Nutrition:

Calories: 481 kcal

Protein: 28.08 g

Fat: 27.52 g

Carbohydrates: 33 g

Avocado and Egg Sandwich

Preparation Time: 10 minutes

Cooking Time: 0 minutes

Servings: 2

Ingredients:

- 1 avocado (ripe)
- 1 egg, organic
- ½ lime juice
- 2 slices of who wheat, seed bread
- 2 radishes
- Black pepper – to your taste
- A pinch of salt (sea or Himalayan)
- 1 scallion
- Mixed seeds – to your choice

Directions:

1. Peel the avocado.
2. Boil the egg (soft boiled).
3. Cut the radishes to thin slices.
4. Dice the scallion (finely).
5. Mix avocado, salt, and lime juice in a bowl. Mash the mixture thoroughly.
6. Spread the mixture onto the bread.
7. Add some radish.

8. Put soft boiled eggs on top.
9. Add some scallion, seeds, and pepper.

Nutrition:

Calories: 342 kcal

Protein: 12.36 g

Fat: 22.99 g

Carbohydrates: 26.54 g

Coconut Porridge

Preparation Time: 20 minutes

Cooking Time: 10 minutes

Servings: 2

Ingredients:

- 2 cups oats
- 1 tbsp. coconut oil
- Coconut milk
- Fresh, shredded coconut (for serving)
- 750 ml of water
- 2 tsp turmeric
- 330ml evaporated coconut milk
- 1 vanilla bean
- 2 tbsp. maple syrup
- 2 tsp ginger
- 1 tsp cinnamon

Directions:

1. Mix 750 ml water and turmeric in a bowl. Let it sit for 10 minutes.
2. Mix all ingredients except coconut milk and shredded coconut in a saucepan.
3. Heat it on medium heat, stirring constantly, and cook for 8 minutes.

4. Let it cool for 10 minutes.
5. Divide into serving bowls.
6. Add coconut milk and shredded coconut on top.
7. Add some extra cinnamon to your taste.
8. Eat warm.

Nutrition:

Calories: 417 kcal

Protein: 20.63 g

Fat: 16.8 g

Carbohydrates: 83.03 g

Almond and Honey Homemade Bar

Preparation Time: 15 minutes + 30 minutes fridge time

Cooking Time: 15 minutes

Servings: 8

Ingredients:

- A ¼ cup of almonds
- 1 cup oats
- ¼ cup sunflower seeds
- 1/3 cup currants
- 1 tbsp. flaxseeds
- 1/3 cup apricots (dried and chopped)
- 1/3 cup raisins (chopped)
- 1 tbsp. sesame seeds
- 1 cup whole-grain puffed cereal (unsweetened)
- ¼ cup almond butter
- ¼ cup honey
- 1/8 tsp salt
- ¼ cup sugar (or another sweetener to your taste in adjusted amount)
- ½ teaspoon vanilla extract

Directions:

1. Preheat the oven to 350 degrees Fahrenheit.
2. Put a baking paper to an 8-inch pan or coat it with cooking spray/oil.
3. Mix the almonds, oats, and seeds and spread the mixture on a rimmed baking sheet.
4. Bake the mixture until you notice that the oats are lightly toasted (for about 10 minutes).
5. Transfer the mixture to a bowl.
6. Add cereal, raisins, currants, and apricots to the bowl.
7. Toss well to combine.
8. Mix honey, almond butter, vanilla, salt, and sugar in a saucepan.
9. Heat over medium heat. Stir frequently for 2-5 minutes until you see light bubbles.
10. As soon as you notice the bubbles, pour the mixture over the dry mixture with apricots and oats you prepared previously.
11. Mix well with a spatula. There mustn't be any dry spots.

12. Transfer the new mixture to the previously prepared pan.
13. Press it to the pan to make a firm and flat layer.
14. Refrigerate for 30 minutes.
15. Cut the layer into eight equal bars or squares, to your taste.
16. Consume immediately or refrigerate up to seven days.
17. You can store these energy bars in the freezer as well (for long-term storage). Wrap them in stretch plastic folium and store at –16 to –18 degrees.

Nutrition:

Calories: 213 kcal

Protein: 6.92 g

Fat: 9.59 g

Carbohydrates: 32.33 g

Desserts

Lemon Vegan Cake

Preparation Time: 10 minutes

Cooking Time: 10 minutes

Servings: 3

Ingredients:

- 1 cup of pitted dates
- 2-1/2 cups pecans
- 1-1/2 cup agave
- 3 avocados, halved & pitted
- 3 cups of cauliflower rice, prepared
- 1 lemon juice and zest
- ½ lemon extract
- 1-1/2 cups pineapple, crushed
- 1-1/2 teaspoon vanilla extract
- Pinch of cinnamon
- 1-1/2 cups of dairy-free yogurt

Directions:

1. Line your baking sheet with parchment paper.
2. Pulse the pecans in your food processor.
3. Add the agave and dates. Pulse for a minute.
4. Transfer this mix to the baking sheet. Wipe the bowl of your processor.
5. Bring together the pineapple, agave, avocados, cauliflower, lemon juice, and zest in your food processor. Get a smooth mixture.
6. Now add the lemon extract, cinnamon, and vanilla extract. Pulse.
7. Pour this mix into your pan, on the crust.
8. Refrigerate for 5 hours minimum.
9. Take out the cake and keep it at room temperature for 20 minutes.
10. Take out the cake's outer ring.
11. Whisk together the vanilla extract, agave, and yogurt in a bowl.
12. Pour on your cake.

Nutrition:

Calories 688

Carbohydrates 100g

Fat 28g

Protein 9g

Sugar 40g

Dark Chocolate Granola Bars

Preparation Time: 10 minutes

Cooking Time: 25 minutes

Servings: 12

Ingredients:

- 1 cup tart cherries, dried
- 2 cups buckwheat
- ¼ cup of flaxseed
- 1 cup of walnuts
- 2 eggs
- 1 teaspoon of salt
- ¼ cup dark cocoa powder
- 2/3 cup honey
- ½ cup dark chocolate chips
- 1 teaspoon of vanilla

Directions:

1. Preheat your oven to 350 degrees F.
2. Apply cooking spray lightly on your baking pan.
3. Pulse together the walnuts, wheat, tart cherries, salt, and flaxseed in your food processor. Everything should be chopped fine.

4. Whisk together the honey, eggs, vanilla, and cocoa powder in a bowl.
5. Add the wheat mix to your bowl. Stir to combine well.
6. Include the chocolate chips. Stir again.
7. Now pour this mixture into your baking dish.
8. Sprinkle some chocolate chips and tart cherries.
9. Bake for 25 minutes. Set aside for cooling before serving.

Nutrition:

Calories 364

Carbohydrates 37g

Cholesterol 60mg

Fat 20g

Protein 6g

Sugar 22g

Fiber 4g

Sodium 214mg

Blueberry Crisp

Preparation Time: 5 minutes

Cooking Time: 30 minutes

Servings: 4

Ingredients:

- ¼ cups pecans, chopped
- 1 cup buckwheat
- ½ teaspoon ginger
- 1 teaspoon of cinnamon
- 2 tablespoons olive oil
- ¼ teaspoon nutmeg
- 1 lb. blueberries
- 1 teaspoon of honey

Directions:

1. Preheat your oven to 350 degrees F.
2. Grease your baking dish.
3. Whisk together the pecans, wheat, oil, spices, and honey in a bowl.
4. Add the berries to your pan. Layer the topping on your berries.
5. Bake for 30 minutes at 350 F.

Nutrition:

Calories 327

Carbohydrates 35g

Fat 19g

Protein 4g

Sugar 14g

Fiber 5g

Sodium 2mg

Potassium 197mg

Chocolate Chip Quinoa Granola Bars

Preparation Time: 5 minutes

Cooking Time: 10 minutes

Servings: 16

Ingredients:

- ½ cup of chia seeds
- ½ cup walnuts, chopped
- 1 cup buckwheat
- 1 cup uncooked quinoa
- 2/3 cup dairy-free margarine
- ½ cup flax seed
- 1 teaspoon of cinnamon
- ½ cup of honey
- ½ cup of chocolate chips
- 1 teaspoon of vanilla
- ¼ teaspoon salt

Directions:

1. Preheat your oven to 350 degrees F.
2. Spread the walnuts, quinoa, wheat, flax, and chia on your baking sheet.
3. Bake for 10 minutes.

4. Line your baking dish with plastic wrap. Apply cooking spray. Keep aside.
5. Melt the margarine and honey in a saucepot.
6. Whisk together the vanilla, salt, and cinnamon into the margarine mix.
7. Keep the wheat mix and quinoa in a bowl. Pour the margarine sauce into it.
8. Stir the mixture. Coat well. Allow it to cool. Stir in the chocolate chips.
9. Spread your mixture into the baking dish. Press firmly into the pan.
10. Plastic wrap. Refrigerator overnight.
11. Slice into bars and serve.

Nutrition:

Calories 408

Carbohydrates 31g

Fat 28g

Protein 8g

Sugar 14g

Fiber 6g

Sodium 87mg

Strawberry Granita

Preparation Time: 10 minutes

Cooking Time: 10 minutes

Servings: 8

Ingredients:

- 2 lb. strawberries, halved & hulled
- 1 cup of water
- Agave to taste
- ¼ teaspoon balsamic vinegar
- ½ teaspoon lemon juice
- Just a small pinch of salt

Directions:

1. Rinse the strawberries in water.
2. Keep in a blender. Add water, agave, balsamic vinegar, salt, and lemon juice.
3. Pulse many times so that the mixture moves. Blend to make it smooth.
4. Pour into a baking dish. The puree should be 3/8 inch deep only.
5. Refrigerate the dish uncovered till the edges start to freeze. The center should be slushy.
6. Stir crystals from the edges lightly into the center. Mix thoroughly.

7. Chill till the granite is almost completely frozen.
8. Scrape loose the crystals like before and mix.
9. Refrigerate again. Use a fork to stir 3-4 times till the granite has become light.

Nutrition:

Calories 72

Carbohydrates 17g

FAT 0G

Sugar 14g

Fiber 2g

Protein 1g

Apple Fritters

Preparation Time: 15 minutes

Cooking Time: 10 minutes

Servings: 4

Ingredients:

- 1 apple, cored, peeled, and chopped
- 1 cup all-purpose flour
- 1 egg
- ½ cup cashew milk
- 1-1/2 teaspoons of baking powder
- 2 tablespoons of stevia sugar

Directions:

1. Preheat your air fryer to 175 degrees C or 350 degrees F.
2. Keep parchment paper at the bottom of your fryer.
3. Apply cooking spray.
4. Mix together ¼ cup sugar, flour, baking powder, egg, milk, and salt in a bowl.
5. Combine well by stirring.
6. Sprinkle 2 tablespoons of sugar on the apples. Coat well.
7. Combine the apples into your flour mixture.

8. Use a cookie scoop and drop the fritters with it to the air fryer basket's bottom.
9. Now air fry for 5 minutes.
10. Flip the fritters once and fry for another 3 minutes. They should be golden.

Nutrition:

Calories 307

Carbohydrates 65g

Cholesterol 48mg

Total Fat 3g

Protein 5g

Sugar 39g

Fiber 2g

Sodium 248mg

Roasted Bananas

Preparation Time: 2 minutes

Cooking Time: 7 minutes

Servings: 1

Ingredients:

- 1 banana, sliced into diagonal pieces
- Avocado oil cooking spray

Directions:

1. Take parchment paper and line the air fryer basket with it.
2. Preheat your air fryer to 190 degrees C or 375 degrees F.
3. Keep your slices of banana in the basket. They should not touch.
4. Apply avocado oil to mist the slices of banana.
5. Cook for 5 minutes.
6. Take out the basket. Flip the slices carefully.
7. Cook for 2 more minutes. The slices of banana should be caramelized and brown. Take them out from the basket.

Nutrition:

Calories 121

Carbohydrates 27g

Cholesterol 0mg

Total Fat 1g

Protein 1g

Sugar 14g

Fiber 3g

Sodium 1mg

Berry-Banana Yogurt

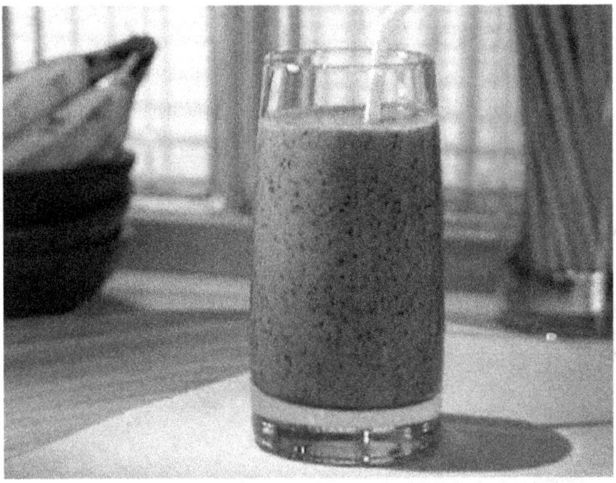

Preparation Time: 10 minutes

Cooking Time: 0 minute

Servings: 1

Ingredients:

- ½ banana, frozen fresh
- 1 container 5.3ounes Greek yogurt, non-fat
- ¼ cup quick-cooking oats
- ½ cup blueberries, fresh and frozen
- 1 cup almond milk
- ¼ cup collard greens, chopped
- 5-6 ice cubes

Directions:

1. Take microwave-safe cup and add 1 cup almond milk and ¼ cup oats
2. Place the cups into your microwave on high for 2.5 minutes
3. When oats are cooked and 2 ice cubes to cool
4. Mix them well
5. Add all ingredients in your blender
6. Blend it until it gets a smooth and creamy mixture
7. Serve chilled and enjoy!

Nutrition:

Calories: 379

Fat: 10g

Carbohydrates: 63g

Protein: 13g

Avocado Chocolate Mousse

Preparation Time: 10 minutes

Cooking Time: 0 minute

Servings: 9

Ingredients:

- 3 ripe avocado, pitted and flesh scooped out
- 6 ounces plain Greek yogurt
- 1/8 cup almond milk, unsweetened
- ¼ cup espresso beans, ground
- ¼ cup of cocoa powder
- ½ teaspoon salt
- 2 tablespoons raw honey
- 1 bar dark chocolate
- 1 teaspoon vanilla extract

Directions:

1. Place all ingredients in your food processor
2. Pulse until smooth
3. Serve chilled and enjoy!

Nutrition:

Calories: 208

Fat: 4g

Carbohydrates: 17g

Protein: 5g

Anti-Inflammatory Apricot Squares

Preparation Time: 20 minutes

Cooking Time: 0 minute

Servings: 8

Ingredients:

- 1 cup shredded coconut, dried
- 1 teaspoon vanilla extract
- 1 cup apricot, dried
- 1 cup macadamia nuts, chopped
- 1 cup apricot, chopped
- 1/3 cup turmeric powder

Directions:

1. Place all ingredients in your food processor
2. Pulse until smooth
3. Place the mixture into a square pan and press evenly
4. Serve chilled and enjoy!

Nutrition:

Calories: 201

Fat: 15g

Carbohydrates: 17g

Protein: 3g

Raw Black Forest Brownies

Preparation Time: 2 hours and 10 minutes

Cooking Time: 0 minute

Servings: 6

Ingredients:

- 1 and ½ cups cherries, pitted, dried and chopped
- 1 cup raw cacao powder
- ½ cup dates pitted
- 2 cups walnuts, chopped
- ½ cup almonds, chopped
- ¼ teaspoon salt

Directions:

1. Place all ingredients in your food processor
2. Pulse until small crumbs are formed
3. Press the brownie batter in a pan
4. Freeze for two hours
5. Slice before serving and enjoy!

Nutrition:

Calories: 294

Fat: 18g

Carbohydrates: 33g

Protein: 7g

Berry Parfait

Preparation Time: 10 min

Cooking Time: 10 min

Servings: 5

Ingredients:

- 7oz / 200g almond butter
- 3.5oz / 100g Greek yogurt
- 14oz / 400g mixed berries
- 2 tsp honey
- 7oz / 200g mixed nuts

Directions:

1. Mix the Greek yogurt, butter, and honey until it's smooth.
2. Add a layer of berries and a layer of the mixture in a glass until it's full.
3. Serve immediately with sprinkled nuts.

Nutrition:

Calories: 250

Carbohydrates: 17 g

Protein: 7.2 g

Fat: 19.4 g

Sugar: 42.3 g

Fiber: 6.6 g, Sodium: 21 mg

Sherbet Pineapple

Preparation Time: 20 Minutes

Cooking Time: 0 Minute

Servings: 4

Ingredients:

- 1 can of 8-ounce pineapple chunks
- 1/3 cup of orange marmalade
- ¼ teaspoon of ground ginger
- ¼ teaspoon of vanilla extract
- 1 can of 11-ounce orange sections
- 2 cups of pineapple, lemon or lime sherbet

Directions:

1. Drain the pineapple, ensure you reserve the juice.
2. Take a medium-sized bowl and add pineapple juice, ginger, vanilla and marmalade to the bowl
3. Add pineapple chunks, drained mandarin oranges as well
4. Toss well and coat everything
5. Free them for 15 minutes and allow them to chill

6. Spoon the sherbet into 4 chilled stemmed sherbet dishes
7. Top each of them with fruit mixture
8. Enjoy!

Nutrition:

Calories: 267 Cal

Fat: 1 g

Carbohydrates: 65 g

Protein: 2 g

Easy Peach Cobbler

Preparation Time: 5 minutes

Cooking Time: 20 minutes

Servings: 6

Ingredients:

- 5 organic peaches, pitted and chopped
- ¼ cup coconut palm sugar, divided
- ½ teaspoon cinnamon
- ¾ cup chopped pecans
- ½ cup gluten-free oats
- ¼ cup ground flaxseeds
- ¼ brown rice flour
- ¼ cup extra virgin olive oil

Directions:

1. Preheat the oven to 3500F.
2. Grease the bottom of 6 ramekins.
3. In a bowl, mix the peaches, ½ of the coconut sugar, cinnamon, and pecans.
4. Distribute the peach mixture into the ramekins.
5. In the same bowl, mix the oats, flaxseed, rice flour, and oil. Add in the remaining

coconut sugar. Mix until a crumbly texture is formed.

6. Top the mixture over the peaches.
7. Place for 20 minutes.

Nutrition:

Calories 26

Fat: 11g

Carbohydrates: 28g

Protein: 10g

Sugar: 12g

Fiber: 6g

Thar She' Salts Peanut Butter Cookies

Preparation Time: 15 Minutes

Cooking Time: 0 0 Minute

Servings: 9

Ingredients:

- 1 cup of raw almonds
- ½ a cup of peanut butter (creamy and unsalted)
- 1 cup of pitted Medjool dates
- 1 and a ¼ teaspoon of vanilla extract
- Sea salt as needed

Directions:

1. Take a food processor and add almonds, peanut butter, vanilla, dates and blend the whole mixture until a dough-like texture comes (should take a few minutes)
2. If you want, add some more peanut butter to make the dough sticker.
3. Form balls using the dough and press down using a fork to create a criss-cross pattern
4. Sprinkle salt generously
5. Serve immediately.

Nutrition:

Calories: 350 Cal

Fat: 17 g

Carbs: 27 g

Protein: 18 g

Almond Butter Balls Vegan

Preparation Time: 10 Minutes

Cooking Time: 0 0 Minute

Servings: 4

Ingredients:

- 12 dates, pitted and diced
- 1/3 cup of unsweetened shredded coconut
- 2 and a ½ tablespoon of almond butter

Directions:

1. Take a bowl and add dates, almond butter, and coconut
2. Mix well
3. Use the mixture to form small balls
4. Store them in your fridge and chill them
5. Enjoy!

Nutrition:

Calories: 62 Cal

Fats: 3 g

Carbohydrates: 8 g

Protein: 1 g

Coffee Cream

Preparation Time: 10 minutes

Cooking Time: 15 minutes

Servings: 4

Ingredients:

- ¼ cup brewed coffee
- 2 tablespoons swerve
- 2 cups heavy cream
- 1 teaspoon vanilla extract
- 2 tablespoons ghee, melted
- 2 eggs

Directions:

1. In a bowl, combine the coffee with the cream and the other ingredients, whisk well and divide it into 4 ramekins and whisk well.
2. Introduce the ramekins in the oven at 350 degrees F and bake for 15 minutes.
3. Serve warm.

Nutrition:

Calories 300

Fat: 11g

Carbohydrates: 3g

Protein: 4g ,Sugar: 12g

Almond Cookies

Preparation Time: 15 min

Cooking Time: 15 min

Servings: 12

Ingredients:

- 14oz / 400g non-wheat flour
- 1tsp baking soda
- 1tsp baking powder
- 3.5oz / 100g tahini
- 1.7oz / 50g coconut butter
- ½ tsp vanilla
- ½ tsp honey
- Salt

Directions:

1. Mix the flour, soda, salt, baking powder together.
2. Mix tahini and coconut butter together and add 2 tbsp. water in the same bowl.
3. Add honey, vanilla to the tahini mixture and blend it well with a mixer.
4. Preheat your oven (180C/356F) and put a baking sheet on it.

5. Add 24 tablespoons of the mixture onto the baking sheet and let it bake in the oven for 11-15 minutes.
6. Let it get cold a little bit and serve.

Nutrition:

Calories: 112

Carbohydrates: 18 g

Protein: 3.2 g

Fat: 1.6 g

Sugar: 23.1 g

Fiber: 7.4 g

Sodium: 28 mg

Chocolate Mousse

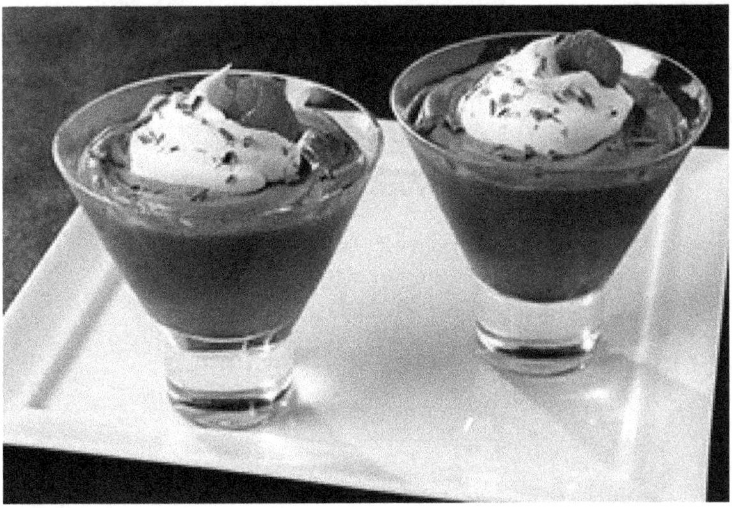

Preparation Time: 10 Minutes

Cooking Time: 0 Minute

Servings: 4

Ingredients:

- Coconut cream scraped from the upper side of 2 pieces of 13.5-ounce chilled cans of full-fat coconut milk
- 4 tablespoons of cocoa
- 3 tablespoons of Agave Nectar
- 1 teaspoon of vanilla extract

Directions:

- Take a large bowl and scoop out the thick coconut cream from the can to the bowl
- Add nectar, vanilla extract and cocoa to the bowl
- Beat it well using an electric mixer, starting from low and going to medium until a foamy texture appears
- Divide the mix evenly amongst ramekins and chill to your desired level of cold
- Enjoy!

Nutrition:

Calories: 134 Cal

Fat: 3.8 g

Carbohydrates: 16 g

Protein: 3.8 g

Raspberry Diluted Frozen Sorbet

Preparation Time: 10 min

Cooking Time: 20 min

Servings: 4

Ingredients:

1. 14oz / 400g frozen raspberry
- 4 fl oz. / 50g almond milk
2. 1 tsp honey
3. Mint

Directions:

- Put the almond milk and raspberry in a mixer till it's smooth and leave the consistency in the freezer for 20 minutes.
- When serving, put them in ice cream bowls and serve with mint on top.

Nutrition:

Calories: 47

Carbohydrates: 11 g

Protein: 1 g

Fat: 0.4 g

Sugar: 37.2 g

Fiber: 6.0 g

Sodium: 24 mg

Chocolate Covered Strawberries

Preparation Time: 15 Minutes

Cooking Time: 0 Minute

Servings: 24

Ingredients:

1. 16 ounces milk chocolate chips
2. 2 tablespoons shortening
3. 1-pound fresh strawberries with leaves

Directions:

- In a bain-marie, melt chocolate and shorter, occasionally stirring until smooth. Hold them by the toothpicks and immerse the strawberries in the chocolate mixture.
- Put toothpicks in the top of the strawberries.
- Turn the strawberries and put the toothpick in the Styrofoam so that the chocolate cools.

Nutrition:

Calories: 115

Cal Fat: 12.5 g

Carbohydrates: 3.2 g

Protein: 6g

Coconut Muffins

Preparation Time: 5 Minutes

Cooking Time: 25 Minutes

Servings: 8

Ingredients:

1. ½ cup ghee, melted
2. 3 tablespoons swerve
3. ¼ teaspoon vanilla extract
4. 1 cup coconut, unsweetened and shredded
5. ¼ cup of cocoa powder
6. eggs, whisked
7. 1 teaspoon baking powder

Directions:

- In a bowl, combine the ghee with the swerve, coconut, and the other ingredients, stir well and divide it into a lined muffin pan. Bake at 370 degrees F for 25 minutes, cool down and serve.

Nutrition:

Calories: 324

Fat: 31g

Carbohydrates: 8.3g

Protein: 4g Sugar: 11g

Chocolate Cherry Chia Pudding

Preparation Time: 4 hours and 5 minutes

Cooking Time: 0 minutes

Servings: 4

Ingredients:

1. 1 ½ cup Any non-dairy milk like coconut or almond milk
2. 3 tbsp. Raw cacao powder
3. ½ cup Sliced pitted cherries
4. ¼ cup Chia seeds you can also use chia seed powder.
5. 3 tbsp. Maple syrup or honey
6. Additional toppings:
7. Raw cacao nibs
8. Extra cherries
9. Dark chocolate shavings (Preferably 70% dark chocolate or more)

Directions:

- Use a mason jar or a bowl. If you're using a bowl, just pour in the milk, maple syrup, chia seeds or powder, and raw cacao. Stir thoroughly and place in the refrigerator for 4 hours or more.

- If you decide to use a mason jar, just pour in the same ingredients, screw the lid on and shake vigorously!
- Serve in separate dishes and top with any or all of the toppings I listed above.
- Enjoy!

Nutrition:

Calories: 811 kcal

Protein: 2.38 g

Fat: 83.36 g

Carbohydrates: 16.88 g

Strawberry Orange Sorbet

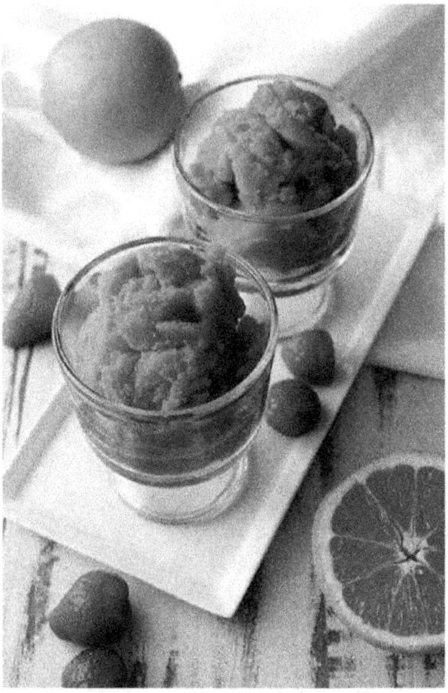

Preparation Time: 5 minutes

Cooking Time: 0 minutes

Servings: 3

Ingredients:

1. 1 cup Orange juice or coconut water
2. 1 pound Frozen strawberries

Direction:

- Pour strawberries in a blender and pulse until all you have left are flakes. 2 minutes tops.

- Now add the coconut water or orange juice and pulse until you get a nice and smooth puree. Have a spatula handy because you might need to scrape some of the puree off the walls of the blender sometimes.
- Serve as soon as you're done or put in the freezer for 45 minutes for a sorbet feel.
- Also, you can pour the smoothie into Popsicle molds and freeze for hours or even overnight.
- Enjoy!

Nutrition:

Calories: 118 kcal

Protein: 2.88 g

Fat: 2.19 g

Carbohydrates: 23.25 g

Pineapple Cake

Preparation Time: 15 minutes

Cooking Time: 50 minutes

Servings: 8

Ingredients:

1. 2 Whole medium eggs
2. 5 tbsp. Raw honey
3. 1 tbsp. Almond flour
4. 1 tsp. Vanilla extract
5. 15 pcs. Frozen sweet cherries
6. 3 tbsp. Melted coconut oil
7. 2 slices Fresh pineapples
8. ½ tsp. Baking powder

Directions:

- Prep oven by preheating to 350°F.
- Remove the skin and core of the pineapples. Set aside.
- Drizzle 1½ tablespoons of raw honey in a round cake tin.
- Layer the pineapple rings and sweet cherries on the honey in a decorative fashion.
- Bring the cake tin in the oven then bake for 15 minutes.

- While all that is going on, mix in the almond and baking powder.
- In a separate bowl, combine the eggs and leftover honey. Drizzle in coconut oil and stir.
- Now add the almond mix to the egg mix and stir thoroughly.
- Take out the cake tin and drizzle batter over the top of the partially baked pineapple rings and use a spatula to spread it evenly.
- Put the cake tin back in the oven and bake for an additional 35 minutes.
- When it's all set, take it out of the oven and leave it to sit for 10 minutes before place it to a plate.
- Serve with extra cherries if you like.

Nutrition:

Calories: 120 kcal

Protein: 2.3 g

Fat: 6.99 g

Carbohydrates: 12.98 g

Mediterranean Rolled Baklava with Walnuts

Preparation Time: 20 minutes

Cooking Time: 40 minutes

Servings: 12

Ingredients:

1. 2 cups Walnuts
2. 1 Lemon zest
3. 1 cup Cream of wheat or plain breadcrumbs
4. 8 sheets Thawed phyllo dough
5. 3 tbsp. Sugar
6. 1/3 cup Milk
7. 3 sticks Melted Unsalted butter
8. Syrup:
9. 1 medium Lemon
10. 3 cups Granulated sugar
11. 3 cups Water

Directions:

- Mix 3 cups of sugar, 3 cups of water and lemon slices in a pan and leave to boil
- Lower the heat, then let it simmer until the sugar completely dissolves. It should take

15 minutes. You should have a nice smooth syrup now. Now leave it to cool for a bit.

- Chop the walnuts in a blender into bits using short pulses.
- Pour the walnuts in a bowl along with the cream of wheat, lemon zest and 4 tablespoons of sugar.
- Stir in milk and set aside.
- Now, preheat your oven to 375°F.
- Spread out the phyllo dough and fit it into a baking pan. Trim off the edges that don't fit with scissors. Cover the remaining phyllo sheets while you work so they don't dry out.
- Place a sheet on a clean flat surface and glaze with melted butter. Do this for all the sheets until it's finished.
- Arrange the walnut mixture on one side of the sheets and roll them up like you're trying to make a sausage. Do this for all the sheets and walnuts.
- Arrange the walnut rolls on an ungreased baking pan and glaze with the leftover butter.

- Bake for about 45 minutes. It's ready when it looks golden.
- Turn off the oven then pull out the baking pan. Drizzle syrup over the baklava, making sure the syrup gets everywhere.
- Bring back the baking pan into the oven then leave to sit for 5 minutes.
- Take off from the oven and leave it to cool for a few hours. Slice the rolls into tiny bits and serve.

Nutrition:

Calories: 488 kcal

Protein: 4.49 g

Fat: 36.89 g

Carbohydrates: 38.21 g

Mint Chocolate Chip Ice-cream

Preparation Time: 5 minutes

Cooking Time: 0 minutes

Servings: 2

Ingredients:

1. 2 Frozen overripe bananas
2. Pinch Spirulina or any natural food coloring, optional.
3. 3 tbsp. Chocolate chips or sugar-free chocolate chips
4. 1/8 tsp. Pure peppermint extract
5. ½ cup raw cashews or coconut cream, optional.
6. Pinch Salt

Directions:

- Mint or imitation peppermint won't be a substitute for this. Use pure peppermint extract and pour it all at once because a drop is more potent than you realize, so add slowly.
- Peel and cut the bananas first. Place the slices in a Ziplock bag then freeze.

- For the ice cream, put all the ingredients in a blender and pulse. You can skip the chocolate chips and just add them after blending. It'll turn out delicious either way.
- Serve as soon as it's ready or freeze until it's firm enough, then serve!

Nutrition:

Calories: 250 kcal

Protein: 6.13 g

Fat: 24.37 g

Carbohydrates: 7.72 g

Flourless Sweet Potato Brownies

Preparation Time: 10 minutes

Cooking Time: 30 minutes

Servings: 9

Ingredients:

1. ½ cup Cooked sweet potato
2. 2 tsp. Vanilla extract
3. ½ cup Almond butter
4. 6 tbsp. Honey
5. ½ tsp. Baking soda
6. 1 large Whole egg
7. ¼ cup Unsweetened Cocoa powder
8. 3 tbsp. Dairy-free chocolate chips, optional.

Directions:

- Prep your oven by preheating to 350°F.
- Line a baking pan with parchment paper leaving a few extra inches on the sides to make it easier to discard or remove
- Blend all the ingredients, excluding the chocolate chips until you get a very smooth and soft batter.

- Transfer the creamy batter to your prepared baking pan and use a spatula to spread it around, so it looks almost even.
- Slide it in the oven, then bake for 30 minutes or until a knife inserted into the pan comes out clean.
- Take off from the oven and leave to cool in the pan for 15 minutes before putting it up on a wire rack.
- If you decide to use the chocolate chip topping, put the chips in a microwave-safe dish and heat until it completely melts. Take off from the microwave and drizzle over the brownies.
- Serve or store!

Nutrition:

Calories: 171 kcal

Protein: 5.17 g

Fat: 9.28 g

Carbohydrates: 20.01 g

Paleo Raspberry Cream Pie

Preparation Time: 20 minutes

Cooking Time: 0 minutes

Servings: 12

Ingredients:

1. For the crust:
2. 1 ½ tbsp. Maple syrup
3. Pinch Salt
4. ½ cup Unsweetened shredded coconut
5. 1 tsp. Vanilla extract
6. 1 cup Roasted or salted cashews
7. Raspberry filling:
8. ¾ cup Unrefined coconut oil
9. 1 ½ cup Roasted or salted cashews
10. ½ cup & 1 tbsp. Maple syrup
11. ¼ cup & 2 tsp. Fresh lemon juice
12. ¼ cup Coconut cream from the top solid part of a can of coconut milk that has been refrigerated overnight
13. 2 tsp. Vanilla extract
14. 3 cups Fresh raspberries
15. Pinch Salt

Directions:

- Prepare 12 muffin pans, line them with muffin liners, and set them aside.
- Make the crust. Set a pan over medium heat and the coconut and stir until it's completely toasted. Stay by the pan because coconuts tend to burn very easily.
- Transfer the toasted coconuts to a bowl and leave to cool for 5 minutes or so. Honestly, this toasting step isn't particularly necessary, but I feel it adds amazing flavor to the crust.
- To make the crust, put all the ingredients in a blender and pulse at the lowest speed until the mix gets all clumpy. Also, don't pulse for too long, or you might end up with a paste. To know if it's ready, put a bit of the mixture on your fingers and pinch. If it gets clumpy, you're on track, if not, add a little water and pulse at the lowest speed for further minutes.
- Scoop the mix into the lined tins using your fingers to pack the mix tightly inside the pan.

- Put the pans to refrigerate while you get to make the filling.
- In a tiny pot set over low heat, stir in all the ingredients until the oil and coconut cream melts completely. Clean the blender using a paper towel and pour in the filling.
- Pulse at high-speed for like 60 seconds or until it's completely smooth. The only clumps we can forgive are the raspberry seeds.
- Drizzle a quarter of the filling over the top of each crust. There should be extra filling; you can store and use that in another dish.
- Place the coated muffins in the fridge to cool. This will take a few hours, like 6 hours, so if you don't have time for that, put it in the freezer.
- To serve, leave them to defrost for 80 minutes or until obviously creamy.

Nutrition:

Calories: 565 kcal

Protein: 7.74 g

Fat: 43.72 g

Carbohydrates: 42.72 g

Caramelized Pears

Preparation Time: 20 minutes

Cooking Time: 5 minutes

Servings: 5

Ingredients:

1. 1 Teaspoon Cinnamon
2. 2 Tablespoon Honey, Raw
3. 1 Tablespoon Coconut Oil
4. 4 Pears, Peeled, Cored & Quartered
5. 2 Cups Yogurt, Plain
6. ¼ Cup Toasted Pecans, Chopped
7. 1/8 Teaspoon Sea Salt

Directions:

- Get out a large skillet, and then heat the oil over medium-high heat.
- Add in your honey, cinnamon, pears, and salt. Cover, and allow it to cook for four to five minutes. Stir occasionally, and your fruit should be tender.
- Uncover it, and allow the sauce to simmer until it thickens. This will take several minutes.

- Soon your yogurt into four dessert bowls. Top with pears and pecans before serving.

Nutrition:

Calories: 290

Protein: 12 Grams

Fat: 11 Grams

Carbs: 41 Grams

Berry Ice Pops

Preparation Time: 3 Hours 5 Minutes

Cooking Time: 0 minutes

Servings: 4

Ingredients:

1. 1 Cup Strawberries, Fresh or Frozen
2. 2 Cups Whole Milk Yogurt, Plain
3. 1 Cup Blueberries, Fresh or Frozen
4. ¼ Cup Water
5. 1 Teaspoon Lemon Juice, Fresh
6. 2 Tablespoons Honey, Raw

Directions:

- Place all together the ingredients in a blender, and blend until smooth.
- Pour into your molds, and freeze for at least three hours before serving.

Nutrition:

Calories: 140

Protein: 5 Grams

Fat: 4 Grams

Carbs: 23 Grams

Fruit Cobbler

Preparation Time: 10 minutes

Cooking Time: 20 minutes

Servings: 8

Ingredients:

1. 1 Teaspoon Coconut Oil
2. ¼ Cup Coconut Oil, Melted
3. 2 Cups Peaches, Fresh & Sliced
4. 2 Cups Nectarines, Fresh & Sliced
5. 2 Tablespoons Lemon Juice, Fresh
6. ¾ Cup Rolled Oats
7. ¾ Cup Almond Flour
8. ¼ Cup Coconut Sugar
9. ½ Teaspoon Vanilla Extract, Pure
10. 1 Teaspoon Ground Cinnamon
11. Dash Salt
12. Filter Water for Mixing

Directions:

- Start by heating your oven to 425.
- Get out a cast-iron skillet, coating it with a teaspoon of coconut oil.
- Mix your lemon juice, peaches, and nectarines together in the skillet.

- Get out a food processor, mixing your almond flour, oats, coconut sugar, and remaining coconut oil. Add in your cinnamon, vanilla, and salt, pulsing until the oat mixture resembles a dry dough.
- If you need more moisture, add filtered water a tablespoon at a time, and then break the dough into chunks, spreading it across the fruit.
- Bake for twenty minutes before serving warm.

Nutrition:

Protein: 4 Grams

Fat: 12 Grams

Carbs: 15 Grams

Watermelon and Avocado Cream

Preparation Time: 2 hours

Cooking Time: 0 minutes

Servings: 4

Ingredients:

1. 2 cups coconut cream
2. 1 watermelon, peeled and chopped
3. 2 avocados, peeled, pitted and chopped
4. 1 tablespoon honey
5. 2 teaspoons lemon juice

Directions:

- In a blender, put all together the ingredients. Divide it into bowls, and keep in the fridge for 2 hours before serving.

Nutrition:

Calories 121

Fat 2

Fiber: 2

Carbs: 6

Protein: 5

Coconut and Chocolate Cream

Preparation Time: 2 hours

Cooking Time: 0 minutes

Servings: 4

Ingredients:

1. 2 cups coconut milk
2. 2 tablespoons ginger, grated
3. 2 tablespoons honey
4. 1 cup dark chocolate, chopped and melted
5. ½ teaspoon cinnamon powder
6. 1 teaspoon vanilla extract

Directions:

- In a blender, put all together the ingredients and blend. Divide into bowls and place in the fridge for 2 hours before serving.

Nutrition:

Calories: 200

Fat: 3

Fiber: 5

Carbs: 12

Protein: 7

Chocolate Bananas

Preparation Time: 5 Minutes

Cooking Time: 15 Minutes

Servings: 4

Ingredients:

1. 3 Bananas, large & cut into thirds
2. 12 oz. Dark Chocolate
3. 1 tbsp. Coconut Oil

Directions:

- Melt the chocolate and coconut oil in a double boiler for 3 to 4 minutes, till you get a smooth and glossy mixture.
- Next, keep the popsicles into the end of each of the banana by inserting it.
- After that, immerse the chocolate into the warm chocolate mixture.
- Shake off the excess chocolate and place them on parchment paper.
- Sprinkle with the topping of your choice.
- Finally, place them in the freezer for a few hours or until set.

- Tip: You can use topping like chopped pistachios or with unsweetened chocolate sprinkles etc.

Nutrition:

Calories: 427Kcal

Proteins: 5.9g

Carbohydrates: 80g

Fat: 15.6g

Watermelon Sorbet

Preparation Time: 5 Minutes

Cooking Time: 15 Minutes

Servings: 4

Ingredients:

1. 1 Seedless Watermelon, cubed

Directions:

- To start with, place the watermelon cubes in a baking sheet in an even layer.
- After that, keep the sheet in the freezer for 2 hours or until the watermelon is solid.
- Next, transfer the frozen watermelon cubes in the high-speed blender and puree them until you get a smooth puree.
- Then, pour the puree among the two loaf pans.

Nutrition:

Calories: 427Kcal

Proteins: 5.9g

Carbohydrates: 80g

Fat: 15.6g

Cinnamon Apple Chips

Preparation Time: 10 Minutes

Cooking Time: 2 Hours

Servings: 3

Ingredients:

2. ¾ tsp. Cinnamon, grounded
3. 3 Honey crisp Apple, large & sweet

Directions:

1. For making this dessert fare, preheat the oven to 200 ° F.
2. After that, keep a parchment paper-lined baking sheet in the middle and lower rack.
3. With the help of an apple corer, core the apples and then slice the apples into 1/8-inch-thick rounds.
4. Then, arrange the apples in the preheated baking sheet in a single layer.
5. Next, sprinkle the cinnamon over the apples.
6. Once sprinkled, bake them for 1 hour.
7. Remove the baking sheet and then switch their position.
8. Bake them for another 1 to 1 ½ hour or until the chips are crispy.

9. Finally, once they are crisp according to your liking, remove the apple chips from the oven.
10. Allow the chips to cool for one hour before serving.
11. Tip: You can top the apple crisps on top of ice creams or yogurt etc.

Nutrition:

Calories: 96Kcal

Proteins: 0g

Carbohydrates: 25.5g

Fat: 0g

Avocado Brownies

Preparation Time: 10 Minutes

Cooking Time: 25 Minutes

Servings: 16

Ingredients:

- 1 tsp. Baking Soda
- 1 Avocado, large
- ¼ tsp. Sea Salt
- ½ cup Applesauce, unsweetened
- ½ cup Cocoa Powder, Dutch-processed & unsweetened
- ½ cup Maple Syrup
- ½ cup Coconut Flour
- 3 Eggs, large
- 1 tap. Vanilla Extract

Directions:

1. First, preheat the oven to 350 ° F.
2. After that, place avocado, vanilla, applesauce, and maple syrup in a high-speed blender and blend for 2 minutes or until smooth.
3. Next, transfer the smooth mixture to a large mixing bowl.

4. To this, stir in the eggs and combine until whisked well.
5. Then, spoon in the coconut flour, sea salt, and cocoa powder to the mixture.
6. Give a good stir until everything comes together.
7. Now, pour the mixture to a greased baking dish and bake for 23 to 25 minutes or until cooked.
8. Lastly, take off from the oven and allow it to cool for 15 to 20 minutes before serving.

Nutrition:

Calories: 91Kcal

Proteins: 1.9g

Carbohydrates: 12.1g

Fat: 4.3g

Fruit Salad

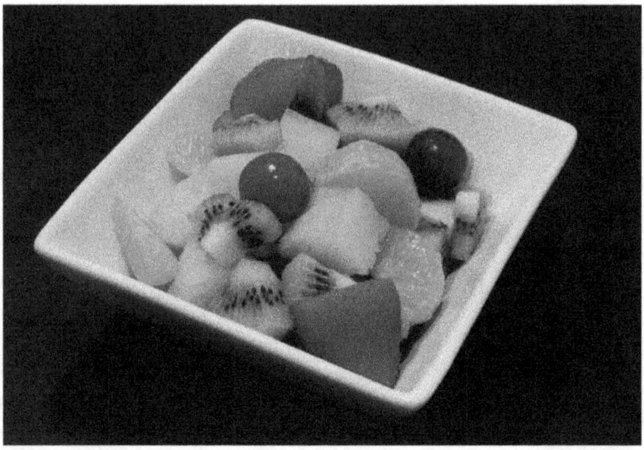

Preparation Time: 10 Minutes

Cooking Time: 20 Minutes

Servings: 2-3

Ingredients:

- ½ of 1 Watermelon, chopped into small pieces
- 1 Pineapple, cut into small pieces
- Dash of Turmeric
- 4 Strawberries, chopped
- 1 Red Papaya, cut into small pieces
- 1 tsp. Ginger, freshly grated
- 1 Pomegranate, small

Directions:

1. To start with, place all the fruits in a large-sized bowl.
2. After that, spoon in the turmeric and ginger over the fruits.
3. Toss well and serve.
4. Tip: Instead of ginger, you can use cinnamon or clove.

Nutrition:

Calories: 118Kcal

Proteins: 1.6g

Carbohydrates: 36.6g

Fat: 0.5g

Chocolate Chip Cookies

Preparation Time: 10 Minutes

Cooking Time: 20 Minutes

Servings: 16

Ingredients:

- ½ cup Maple Syrup
- 2 cups Almond Flour, finely sifted
- ½ cup Almond Butter
- ½ cup Dark Chocolate Chips, sugar-free

Directions:

1. Preheat the oven to 350 ° F.
2. Next, combine the almond flour, almond butter, and maple syrup in a medium-sized mixing bowl until mixed well.
3. To this, stir in the chocolate chips and mix again.
4. With the help of an ice cream scooper, scoop out the mixture to a greased baking sheet. Flatten the top slightly with your hand.
5. Finally, bake them for 10 to 12 minutes or until they are going to get browned.

Nutrition:

Calories: 176Kcal

Proteins: 5g

Carbohydrates: 16g

Fat: 11g

Conclusion

The anti-inflammatory diet cookbook is the perfect resource for anyone who is suffering from inflammation. This cookbook has a special focus on reducing inflammation in the joints, cartilage, and muscles. Each recipe has been carefully developed to help reduce joint pain, joint stiffness, and even autoimmune disorders such as lupus and rheumatoid arthritis.

While most people associate food with comfort, a large number of foods are actually capable of having a dramatic impact on your health. Foods that are high in good fats (omega-3) are especially beneficial for many issues that affect the body. This cookbook provides recipes that are high in good fats and low in inflammatory foods like gluten and dairy. These recipes can be used to help create an anti-inflammatory diet that can help you feel better! The inflammatory disease will lead to many different health consequences and will even attack our most vital organs. The best way to do this is to prevent chronic inflammation in the first place. The next best thing is to recognize the signs and symptoms as early as possible, so proper interventions can be done to limit and reverse the impact of chronic inflammation. Inflammatory disease is the root cause of many long-term diseases, so ignoring the warning signs can create major consequences for your health.

Unfortunately, if the inflammatory disease gets out of control, preventative measures may be out of the question, and medical interventions will need to be done. Our goal is to prevent you from getting to this point. Lucky for us, many lifestyle changes can be performed to stop and reverse this disease process when it is still in its in advance stages. This is another reason why we should recognize and not ignore the signs and symptoms. A major lifestyle change we can commit to is a new diet plan. The anti-inflammatory diet is a meal plan that boasts healthy and nutritious cuisines, but still flavorful and appealing to the taste buds. There is a major myth out there that healthy food cannot be delicious. We have proven this myth wrong by providing numerous recipes from around the world that follow our healthy meal plan.

We hope that the information you read in this book gives you a better understanding of how the immune system functions and how a proper diet plan can help protect it and our other valuable cells and tissues. The recipes we have provided are just a starting point. Use them as a guide to create many of your dishes that follow the diet plan. Just make sure you use the proper ingredients and food groups. Also, for maximum results, follow the Anti-Inflammatory Diet food Guide Pyramid.

The next step is to take the instruction we have provided and begin taking steps to change your life and improve your health. Begin recognizing the signs and symptoms of chronic inflammation and make the necessary lifestyle changes to prevent further health problems. Start transitioning to the anti-inflammatory diet today by incorporating small meals into your schedule and increase the amount as tolerated. Within a short period, the diet will be a regular part of your routine. You will notice increased energy, improved mental function, a stronger and well-balanced immune system, reduction in chronic pain, some healthy weight loss, and overall better health outcomes. If you are ready to experience these changes, then wait no longer and begin putting your knowledge from this book into action.

CPSIA information can be obtained
at www.ICGtesting.com
Printed in the USA
BVHW092238260421
605884BV00008B/145

9 781801 836814